RADICAL WEIGHT REDUCTION

Everything you need to know about weight loss

Dr Bertil E. Lindmark, MD, PhD

RADICAL WEIGHT REDUCTION

Desperate to lose weight?

Tired of being fat?

Everything you need to know about weight loss in one book!

Table of content:

Introduction

Most people find it very difficult if not impossible to lose weight.

Actually, both the access to food, modern housing and means of transportation leads to more intakes and less energy expenditure.

Your brain is set in a mode that actually prevents you from losing weight. Therefore, losing weight is extremely difficult, but not impossible.

This book will give you all the information you need to lose weight, from understanding how our body functions, to methods for weight loss.

If you are tired of being fat, then start reading!

Chapter 1: Why should you lose weight

Overweight is for most people with moderate fatness, a problem of appearance. Importantly though, and as most people know, overweight is linked to a large number of health issues.

The problem of overweight is not a rational one. Most of us understand and agree the arguments and understand the basis of our inability to reduce weight, but the mechanisms that work against our best resolution are too strong.

Therefore, this book tries to answer the question - how do we need to behave to reduce weight and to overpower the forces that make us grow and keep us fat?

If you really want to lose weight, there are several steps you need to consider, from natural weight reduction, through medicines and even surgery.

But before you can lose weight, you need to learn the basis of weight loss!

Chapter 2: Simple understanding of weight loss

In theory, losing weight is easy. The primary factor that determines whether you gain or lose weight is your caloric intake (how many calories you eat).

If you eat more calories than you burn (hypercaloric diet), you will gain weight and if you burn more calories than you eat (hypocaloric diet), you will lose weight.

When you eat exactly the same amount of calories as you burn, it is called a maintenance caloric diet.

So, if you maintain your current body weight consuming 2200 calories per day (this would be your "maintenance level"), you'd lose weight if you burn more than 2200 calories.

But the reality is something else.

Our bodies react differently to the amount of foods that we eat and the activities that we partake in, therefore we require customized approaches. There are weight loss calculators & tools that we can use to establish the status of our bodies and what we need to do to lose weight and monitor our progress as we go.

Tools and calculators are great motivators, it allows you to track the progress of your program at any time and helps you focus on your goals.

Weight Loss Calculators & Tools

Calories Required To Lose Weight Calculator

The Calorie calculator allows you to calculate how many calories you require daily, in order to lose a certain amount of weight within a certain time period.

Calorie Counter (Food)

The calorie counter will help you determine the calorie count for many calories in food, including fast food calories, calories in fruit and calories in restaurant food.

Body Mass Index Calculator

Use the body mass index calculator to calculate your body mass index (BMI).

Calorie Activity Calculator

Use the calorie calculator to find out how many calories you burn for over 70 activities and exercises.

Online Diary

Use the free online diary where you can jot down any of your thoughts about absolutely anything.

Weight tracker

The personal weight tracker allows you to track the progress of your weight, your result is represented with a bar graph and table.

Chapter 3: Natural weight loss

Natural weight loss is the best way to lose weight. It should **ALWAYS** be the first step!

Changing the bad habits

It is very clear that if you eat 2 pizzas per day and you never do exercise, you are likely to get morbidly fat.

So, what can you do?

Most of us are creatures of habit. We buy the same foods from the same grocery store and prepare the same recipes over and over. If you're serious about eating healthier and losing weight, you need to shake it up, change those bad eating habits, and start thinking differently about your diet and lifestyle.

The problem is that we get so comfortable in our ways that it's hard to give up those old habits. Even when you want to change, old habits die hard.

Even those who manage to change their bad eating habits can easily fall back on their old ways during times of stress. When you're feeling weak or vulnerable, automatic responses often override good intentions.

Tackling bad eating and exercise habits require a three-pronged approach:

- Being aware of the bad habits you want to fix.

- Figuring out why these habits exist.

- Eating a healthier diet may be intimidating at first. But once you see for yourself how good it makes you feel, and how good healthy food can taste, you have a better chance of succeeding.

You're much more likely to be successful at changing your habits if you take things one step at a time. Try to gradually incorporate new habits over time, and before you know it, you will be eating more healthfully and losing weight.

Eating a healthier diet may be intimidating at first. But once you see for yourself how good it makes you feel and how good healthy food can taste, you have a better chance of succeeding. Over time, your preferences will change and cravings for bad foods will fade away.

4 Steps to Fix Bad Eating Habits

1. Take Baby Steps:

- Making small changes in your diet and lifestyle can improve your health, as well as trim your waistline.

- Start each day with a nutritious breakfast.

- Get 8 hours of sleep each night, as fatigue can lead to overeating.

- Eat your meals seated at a table, without distractions.

- Eat more meals with your partner or family.

- Teach yourself to eat when you're really hungry and stop when you're comfortably full.

- Reduce your portion sizes by 20%, or give up second helpings.

- Try lower-fat dairy products.

- Make sandwiches with whole-grain bread and spread them with mustard instead of mayo.

- Eat a nutritious meal or snack every few hours.

- Try different cooking methods, such as grilling, roasting, baking, or poaching.

- Drink more water and fewer sugary drinks.

- Eat smaller portions of calorie-dense foods (like casseroles and pizza) and larger portions of water-rich foods (like broth-based soups, salads, and veggies).

- Limit alcohol to 1-2 drinks per day.

2. Become More Mindful:

- One of the first steps toward conquering bad eating habits is paying more attention to what you're eating and drinking. Read food labels, become familiar with lists of ingredients, and start to take notice of everything you put into your mouth. Once you become more aware of what you're eating, you'll start to realize how you need to improve your diet.

3. Make a Plan:

- How are you going to start eating more fruit, having breakfast every day, or getting to the gym more often? Spell out your options. For example: Plan to take a piece of fruit to work every day for snacks, stock up on cereal and fruit for quick breakfasts, and go to the gym on the way to work three times a week.

4. Be Realistic:

- Don't expect too much from yourself too soon. It takes about a month for any new action to become habit.

5. Tackle a New Mini-Goal Each Week:

These mini-steps will eventually add up to major change. For example, if your goal is to eat more vegetables, tell yourself you'll try one new veggie each week until you find some you really enjoy. Or look for easy ways to add one more serving of vegetables to your diet each week, until you reach your goal. You can try topping your lunch sandwich with slices of cucumbers; adding shredded carrots to the muffins you have for breakfast…

Trick Your Brain Into Eating Less

Like most things in life, losing weight is in large part of mind over matter. Whether or not you realize it your mind, and how you think about food has a lot to do with whether or not you will lose weight. While having a positive mind set and realistic weight loss goals will help you to achieve your goals, there are other ways to trick your mind and your body into eating less which ultimately will result in weight loss.

Here are some tricks you can use to help fool your mind into helping your body lose weight:

Don't Diet:

The moment you mention or even think the word diet, a list of negative connotations go through your subconscious. Your conscious mind may be thinking weight loss, but your subconscious mind is thinking, deprivation, hunger, and suffering. Forget about dieting and focus your mind on eating healthier.

Don't Bring Serving Bowls To The Table:

Even if your body feels sated with the food on your plate, seeing bowls with food still in them, often signals your mind that you need to eat more food. Perhaps, this is due to the fact that your mother has burned into your mind that you should not waste food, or that you need to finish a small portion left in a bowl so the bowl can be washed. Whatever, the reason, seeing food remain in a serving bowl, makes us reach for more, even when we are not longer hungry.

Sticking To Portion Size While Filling The Plate:

Believe it or not, starting out with a filled plate at a meal, actually can help you to eat less. Many times your brain simply signals that you need to eat more when your plate has too much white space. However, you can trick your brain into seeing more food than is actually there simply by placing those smaller portions on a smaller plate or one with a large rim. When your plate looks full, you actually think you are eating more.

Chew Eat Bite 20 Times:

Not only chewing your food will help you digest it better, but it also has both a physical impact and a mental one on how full you feel. Physically, when you eat your food quickly, your body does not have a chance to start digesting what you are eating, so you eat more because you don't feel full. By eating more slowly your body has a chance to feel sated, and therefore you tend to eat less.

Eating fast also has a physiological impact on how full you feel. When you eat slowly it takes more time to finish a meal and the longer you eat, the more likely your mind will think you have eaten a large quantity of food. You feel like you have eaten more simply because your body tells you that you have.

Choose Foods With A Lot Of Color:

Believe it or not, the more colorful that plate of food is, the more full you may feel. Eating a monochromatic plate of food leaves most people feeling unsatisfied, so they tend to eat more.

So go ahead and eat that chicken breast, but try placing it on a dark green leaf of Kale and a slice or two of orange or lemon. Throw some broccoli and carrots in with that ½ cup of brown rice to make it more visually appealing and enjoy a side of fresh raspberries or blueberries. By making your plate of food more colorful, not only do you feel like you have eaten more, but you are actually taking in wider variety of vitamins, minerals, and other nutrients all of which make you feel fuller.

Sit Down At A Table To Eat Your Meal or Snack:

One of the tricks that your mind plays on you is telling you that any food you consume while watching television, sitting at a computer, or lounging on the couch or bed simply do not count. So, you tend to think of food you eat in these places as not being real meals, and therefore your mind tells you that you need something more. By sitting down at a table and making the act of eating, an activity in itself, you become more aware of just how much food you are consuming and are likely to eat less.

Tricking your mind into helping your body eat less while feeling more satisfied will help you to reach those weight loss goals much faster while feeling less hungry. Much of the weight loss process is truly mind over matter.

Fool your brain - fat instead of carbs

Carbohydrates are excellent sources of energy, but start a process in which you get blood sugar swings up and then down; that will make you hungry.

When you get hungry, you end up looking for fast reduction of hunger, so you eat more carbs.

And so it goes / do you get it?

Instead of having a lot of carbs, a fat based diet is more likely to reduce the vicious circle and get you stable. There are many low carb diets (you can find it on Google), but basically it is about fooling your brains by eating fat, especially small amounts of fat and preventing hunger.

Get more exercise

One of the biggest reasons we have weight problems is the fact that we are sitting too much. Adults should be involved in at least 150 minutes of moderate activity or 75 minutes of some exercise activity each week, or a combination of these two. Young children must engage at least an hour of some vigorous activity per day, in order to improve their cardiovascular and physical health. You should avoid or at least limit all sedentary activities, such as playing games on the computer.

By exercising on a daily basis, you`ll not only lose weight, but also it will prevent many health conditions.

Simple Ways to Move Your Body

- Once a week, turn off the TV and do something a little more physical with your family. Play games, take a walk; almost anything will be more active than sitting on the couch.

- Look for small ways to walk more. When you get the mail, take a walk around the block or take the dog for a walk.

- Do some chores; working in the garden, raking leaves, sweeping the floor - these kinds of activities may not be 'vigorous' exercise, but they can keep you moving while getting your house in order.

- Pace while you talk; when you're on the phone, pace around. This is a great way to stay moving while doing something you enjoy.

Diets

With over 1,000 diet books available, popular diets have clearly become increasingly prevalent. At the same time, they have also become increasingly controversial, because some depart substantially from mainstream medical advice or have been criticized by various medical authorities.

The truth is that sticking with a diet (more than the type of a diet), is the key to losing weight.

Unfortunately, most weight-loss diets are hard to stick to long enough to reach your weight goal. And some may not be healthy. Diets that leave you feeling deprived or hungry may create irresistible cravings — or worse yet, may leave you feeling like giving up. And because most weight-loss diets don't encourage permanent healthy lifestyle changes, the pounds you do lose often quickly come back once you stop dieting.

Successful weight loss requires permanent changes to your eating habits and physical activity. This means you need to find a weight-loss approach that you can embrace for life. Even then, you may always have to remain vigilant about your weight. But combining a healthier diet and more activity is the best way to lose weight and keep it off for the long term.

Before starting a weight-loss program, talk to your doctor about weight-loss plans you may have tried before and what you liked or didn't like about them.

Consider your personal needs

There's no single weight-loss diet that will help everyone who tries it. But if you consider your preferences, lifestyle and weight-loss goals, you should be able to find or tailor a diet to suit your individual needs. Before starting another weight-loss program, think about these factors:

Your experience with past diets:

Think about diets you may have tried before. What did you like or dislike about them? Were you able to follow the diet? What worked or didn't work for you? How did you feel physically and emotionally while on the diet?

Your preferences:

Do you prefer to diet on your own, or do you like getting support from a group? If you like group support, do you prefer online support or in-person meetings?

Your budget:

Some weight-loss programs require you to buy supplements or meals, or to visit weight-loss clinics or attend support meetings. Does the cost of such programs fit your budget?

Other considerations:

Do you have a health condition, such as diabetes, heart disease or allergies? Do you have specific cultural or ethnic requirements or preferences when it comes to food? These are important factors that should help determine which diet you choose.

Successful weight loss requires a long-term commitment to making healthy changes in your eating and exercise habits. Be sure to pick an eating plan you can live with. Look for a plan with these features:

Flexible:

Look for a plan that doesn't forbid certain foods or food groups, but instead includes a variety of foods from all the major food groups. A healthy diet includes vegetables and fruits, whole grains, low-fat dairy products, lean protein sources, and nuts and seeds — and even an occasional sweet indulgence. A diet plan should also feature foods that you can easily find in your local grocery store.

Balanced:

A weight-loss plan should include proper amounts of nutrients and calories for your individual situation. Diets that direct you to eat large quantities of certain foods, such as grapefruit or meat, that drastically cut calories, or that eliminate entire food groups, such as carbohydrates, may result in nutritional problems. Safe diets do not require excessive vitamins or supplements.

Chapter 4: The Radical Alternatives

If you have tried all of the natural ways to lose weight and failed, then it is time for alternatives!

Medicine

(Brand names will differ in different markets!)

There are several medicines that can help you cheat and fool your brain. Most only have a modest influence on your weight. The principles are to reduce fat uptake from the gut, stimulate calorie consumption, or reduce the hunger signals.

To get access you need to have a prescription. And obviously, as with all medicines, there are both risks for side effects and risk of no effect. If you have serious health problems because of your weight and dieting hasn't worked for you, prescription weight-loss drugs may be an option.

Weight loss drugs like Xenical and Meridia do exist and also work. Their effects are modest, usually resulting in a loss of no more than 10% of a person's body weight. Contrary to some hopes, they don't replace diet and exercise; weight loss drugs only work in conjunction with lifestyle changes.

You'll still need to focus on diet and exercise while taking these drugs, and they're not for everyone.

Doctors usually prescribe them only if your BMI is 30 or higher, or if it's at least 27 and you have a condition that may be related to your weight, like type 2 diabetes or high blood pressure.

Here's what you should know about four of the most common prescriptions for weight loss:

Orlistat:

How it works: Blocks your body from absorbing about a third of the fat you eat. When a doctor prescribes Orlistat, it's called Xenical. If you get it without a prescription, it's called Alli, which has half of Xenical's dose.

Approved for long-term use? Yes.

Side effects: Abdominal cramping, passing gas, leaking oily stool, having more bowel movements, and not being able to control bowel movements. These side effects are generally mild and temporary. But they may get worse if you eat high-fat foods. Rare cases of severe liver injury have been reported in people taking Orlistat, but it's not certain that the drug caused those problems.

What else you should know: You should be on a low-fat diet (less than 30% of your daily calories from fat) before taking Orlistat. Take a multivitamin at least 2 hours before or after taking Orlistat, because the drug temporarily makes it harder for your body to absorb vitamins A, D, E, and K.

Belviq:

How it works: Curbs your appetite.

Approved for long-term use? Yes.

Side effects in people who don't have diabetes: headache, dizziness, nausea, fatigue, dry mouth, and constipation. The most common side effects in those who have diabetes: low blood sugar (hypoglycemia), headache, back pain, cough and fatigue.

What else you should know: If you don't lose 5% of your weight after 12 weeks of taking Belviq, you should stop taking it, because it's unlikely to work for you.

Phentermine:

How it works: Curbs your appetite. Your doctor may prescribe this under the names Apidex or Suprenza.

Approved for long-term use? No. It's approved for short-term use (a few weeks) only.

Side effects: Raised blood pressure or heart palpitations, restlessness, dizziness, tremor, insomnia, shortness of breath, chest pain, and trouble doing activities you've been able to do. Phentermine may make you drowsy, hampering your ability to drive or operate machinery. As with some other appetite suppressants, there's a risk of becoming dependent upon the drug.

Don't take it late in the evening, as it may cause insomnia. You should not take phentermine if you have a history of, heart disease, stroke, congestive heart failure, or uncontrolled high blood pressure. You also shouldn't take it if you have glaucoma or a history of drug abuse, or if you are pregnant or nursing.

What else you should know: Phentermine is an amphetamine. Because of the risk of addiction or abuse, such stimulant drugs are "controlled substances," which means they need a special type of prescription.

Qsymia:

How it works: Curbs your appetite.

Approved for long-term use? Yes.

Side effects: Tingling hands and feet, dizziness, altered sense of taste, insomnia, constipation, and dry mouth. Serious side effects include certain birth defects (cleft lip and cleft palate), faster heart rate, suicidal thoughts or actions, and eye problems that could lead to permanent vision loss, if not treated.

You shouldn't take Qsymia if you have glaucoma, hyperthyroidism, heart disease, or stroke. Get regular checks of your heart when starting the drug or increasing the dose.

What else you should know: If you don't lose 3% of your weight after 12 weeks on Qsymia, you stop taking it.

Supplements

With all the new weight loss medications entering the market, many people are also looking for supplements to aid weight loss.

Hydroxycitrate, Hydroxycitric Acid or HCA:

HCA is actually a salt derived from the rind of dried fruit, in particular the Southeast Asian plants brindall berry and Garcinia Cambodia. It's sold in drug stores and supplement stores as HCA, brindleberry or brindall berry and garcinia. Research backs the effectiveness of HCA at reducing fat absorption, increasing fat metabolism, inhibiting appetite, and lowering LDL cholesterol.

Chitosan:

Chitosan is recommended by wholistic practitioners to lower cholesterol and it has also been promoted as a type of dietary fiber that may help reduce the absorption of fat.

Whey protein:

Weight protein is known as a muscle builder; however, it also suppresses appetite, thus helping you eat less. Whey protein is an easily digestible form of protein. It contains high levels of the amino acid cysteine.

Beta Glucan

A concentrated soluble fiber derived from yeasts, mushrooms, and algae, beta-glucans comes in many forms, but all have the effect of lowering cholesterol with the additional benefits of weight loss and helping control diabetes.

Conjugated Linoleic Acid or CLA

CLA is found primarily in beef and dairy products, so if you're vegetarian or vegan, you likely aren't getting enough. CLA is one of the more popular health food supplements for reduction of body fat, though the evidence is mixed. Animal studies have shown it to be effective, but human studies have been mixed.

Glucomannan

Derived from an Asian plant called Konjac, glucomannan is a fiber considered extremely effective for diabetes and blood sugar control, with the additional properties of weight loss. The fiber helps absorb water in the digestive tract, reducing cholesterol and carbohydrate absorption, and research supports its role as an obesity treatment.

Mango Seed Fiber

Fiber from the seeds of the African mango tree is a traditional African weight loss remedy that's finding new popularity either alone or combined with other dietary supplements. It's most commonly used in Africa as a natural antibiotic and pain reliever. It's currently being studied for weight loss, diabetes and cholesterol reduction.

Not recommended alternatives

Smoking

Smoking increases energy expenditure by 15% (and obviously does a lot of harm to your body – lungs, skin, bone lose out and the risk for cancer goes up by 30%).

Smoking also reduces hunger signals. It is very addictive, so if you start, it stays with you like something unwanted on the sole of your shoe.

Drugs (Illegal)

Amphetamine and cocaine are known to cause weight reduction. They reduce hunger and cause physical over-activity.

Human growth hormone is another medicine, which has been used as an illicit means to reduce weight.

Obviously, narcotics and off-label use of drugs is prohibited by law and are physically dangerous, and can therefore not be recommended!

I strongly recommend not to use drugs and tobacco!

Chapter 5: Getting Radical

- If you have tried everything (diets, exercises, medicine), and none of that have worked, then you should consider some more radical solutions.

Surgery

Weight loss surgery, also called bariatric surgery, is used as a last resort to treat people who are dangerously obese (carrying an abnormally excessive amount of body fat).

This type of surgery is only available for people with potentially life-threatening obesity when other treatments, such as lifestyle changes, haven't worked.

Potentially life-threatening obesity is defined as:

- Having a body mass index (BMI) of 40 or above

- Having a BMI of 35 or above and having another serious health condition that could be improved if you lose weight, such as type 2 diabetes or high blood pressure

For people who meet the above criteria, weight loss surgery has proved to be effective in significantly and quickly reducing excess body fat.

Surgical methods to reduce weight

Deciding to get weight loss surgery isn't easy, and after making the decision to do it, there are still many different procedures to choose from. The best surgery for an individual is based on a lot of criteria: your goals, surgeon's preference, current health, and of course, which procedures are covered by your insurance.

Choosing a specific surgical approach will require a lot of thought and discussion with your doctor. There are two basic types of weight loss surgery - restrictive surgeries and malabsorptive/restrictive surgeries. They help with weight loss in different ways.

Restrictive surgeries work by physically restricting the size of the stomach and slowing down digestion. A normal stomach can hold about 3 pints of food. After surgery, the stomach may at first hold as little as an ounce, although later that could stretch to 2 or 3 ounces. The smaller the stomach, the less you can eat. The less you eat, the more weight you lose.

Malabsorptive/restrictive surgeries are more invasive surgeries that work by changing how you take your food. In addition to restricting the size of the stomach, these surgeries physically remove or bypass parts of your digestive tract, which makes it harder for your body to absorb calories. Purely malabsorptive surgeries, also called intestinal bypasses, are no longer done because of the side effects.

Specific Types of Weight Loss Surgery

Surgery has its own risks and obviously you will need to discuss which method is best for you. Some methods are non-invasive which means that you do not need to reach the stomach through cutting through your skin, and therefore may carry less risk.

Adjustable Gastric Banding:

Gastric banding is among the least invasive weight loss treatments. This surgery uses an inflatable band to squeeze the stomach into two sections: a smaller upper pouch and a larger lower section. The two sections are still connected; the channel between them is very small, which slows down the emptying of the upper pouch. Gastric banding physically restricts the amount of food you can take in per meal. Most people can only eat ½ to 1 cup of food before feeling too full or sick. The food also needs to be soft or well-chewed.

Pros: The advantage of gastric banding is that it's simpler to do and safer than gastric bypass and other operations. It's routinely done as minimally invasive surgery, using small incisions, special instruments, and a tiny camera called a laparoscope. Recovery is usually faster. You can also have it reversed by surgically removing the band. Because the band is connected to an opening just beneath the skin in the abdomen, it can be easily loosened or tightened in the doctor's office.

Cons: People who get gastric band often have less dramatic weight loss than those who get more invasive surgeries. They may also be more likely to regain some of the weight over the years.

Risks: The most common side effect of gastric banding is vomiting, a result of eating too much too quickly. Complications with the band aren't uncommon. It might slip out of place, or become too loose, or leak. Sometimes, further surgeries are necessary. As with any surgery, infection is always a risk. Although unlikely, some complications can be life-threatening.

Sleeve Gastrectomy:

Sleeve Gastrectomy is another form of restrictive weight loss surgery. In the operation, which is usually done with a laparoscope, about 75% of the stomach is removed. What remains of the stomach is a narrow tube or sleeve, which connects to the intestines. Sometimes, a sleeve gastrectomy is a first step in a sequence of weight loss surgeries. It can be followed up by gastric bypass or biliopancreatic diversion, if more weight loss is needed. However, in other cases, it might be the only surgery you need.

Pros: For people who are very obese or sick, standard gastric bypass or biliopancreatic diversion may be too risky. A sleeve gastrectomy is a simpler operation that allows them a lower-risk way to lose weight. If needed, once they've lost weight and their health has improved - usually after 12 months to 18 months, they can have a second surgery, such as gastric bypass. People with high BMIs result in an average weight loss of greater than 50% of excess weight.

Because the intestines aren't affected, a sleeve gastrectomy doesn't affect the absorption of food, so nutritional deficiencies are not a problem.

Cons: Unlike gastric banding procedures, a sleeve gastrectomy is irreversible. Most importantly, since it's relatively new, the long-term benefits and risks are still being evaluated.

Risks: Typical surgical risks include infection, leaking of the sleeve, and blood clots.

Gastric Bypass Surgery:

Gastric bypass is the most common type of weight loss surgery. It combines both restrictive and malabsorptive approaches. It can be done as either a minimally invasive or open surgery. In the operation, the surgeon divides the stomach into two parts, sealing off the upper section from the lower. The surgeon then connects the upper stomach directly to the lower section of the small intestine. Essentially, the surgeon is creating a shortcut for the food, bypassing a section of the stomach and the small intestine. Skipping these parts of the digestive tract means that fewer calories get absorbed into the body.

Pros: Weight loss tends to be swift and dramatic. About 50% of it happens in the first six months. It may continue for up to two years after the operation. Because of the rapid weight loss, health conditions affected by obesity, such as diabetes, high blood pressure, often improve quickly. You'll probably also feel dramatic improvements in your quality of life. Gastric bypass also has good long-term results; studies have found that many people keep most of the weight off for 10 years or longer.

Cons: By design, surgeries like this impair the body's ability to absorb food. While that can cause rapid weight loss, it also puts you at risk of serious nutritional deficiencies. The loss of calcium and iron could lead to osteoporosis and anemia.
You'll have to be very careful with your diet and take supplements for the rest of your life. Unlike adjustable gastric banding, gastric bypass is generally considered irreversible. It has been reversed in rare cases. Therefore, getting this surgery means that

you're permanently changing how your body digests food.

Gastric bypass surgery can lead to a dumping syndrome, in which food is "dumped" from the stomach into the intestines too quickly, before it's been properly digested. About 85% of people who get a gastric bypass have some dumping. Symptoms include nausea, bloating, pain, sweating, weakness and diarrhea. Dumping is often triggered by sugary or high-carbohydrate foods and adjusting your diet helps. However, some experts actually see dumping syndrome as beneficial, because it encourages people to avoid foods that could lead to weight gain.

Risks: Because these weight loss surgeries are more complicated, the risks are higher. The risk of death from these procedures is low, about 1% - but they are more dangerous than gastric banding. Infection and blood clots are risks, as they are with most surgeries. Gastric bypass also increases the risk of hernias, which can develop later and may need further surgery to fix. Also, a side effect of rapid weight loss can be the formation of gallstones.

Biliopancreatic Diversion:

Biliopancreatic Diversion is essentially a more drastic version of a gastric bypass, in which part of the stomach, as much as 70%, is removed and even more of the small intestine is bypassed. A somewhat less extreme version of this weight loss surgery is called biliopancreatic diversion with a duodenal switch or "the duodenal switch." While still more involved than a gastric bypass, this procedure removes less of the stomach and bypasses less of the small intestine. It also reduces the risk of dumping syndrome, malnutrition, and ulcers, which are more common with a standard biliopancreatic diversion.

Pros: Biliopancreatic diversion can result in even greater and faster weight loss than a gastric bypass. Studies show an average long-term loss of 70% to 80% of excess weight. Although much of the stomach is removed, the remainder is still larger than the pouches formed during gastric bypass or banding procedures. So you may actually be able to eat larger meals with this surgery than with others.

Cons: Biliopancreatic diversion is less common than gastric bypass. One of the reasons is that the risk of nutritional deficiencies is much serious. It also poses many of the same risks as gastric bypass, including dumping syndrome. However, the duodenal switch may lower some of these risks.

Risks: This is one of the most complicated and high-risk weight loss surgeries. According to National Institutes of Health, the risk of death from the duodenal switch ranges between 2.5% and 5%. As with gastric bypass, this surgery poses a fairly high risk of hernia, which will need further surgery to correct.

So which weight loss surgery is the best?

The ideal weight loss surgery depends on your current health and body type. For instance, if you are very obese, or had abdominal surgery before, minimally invasive surgeries might not be possible. It really pays to talk with your doctor about the pros and cons of each procedure.

If possible, go to a medical center that specializes in weight loss surgery. Studies have shown that the risk of complications is lower when weight loss surgery is done by experts.

No matter where you are, always make sure that your surgeon has had plenty of experience performing the procedure you need.

Benefits and Risks of Weight Loss Surgery

Weight loss surgery is a serious undertaking. Before making a decision, talk to your doctor about the following benefits and risks.

Benefits

Weight loss: Immediately following surgery, most patients lose weight rapidly and continue to do so until 18 to 24 months after the procedure. Although most patients then start to regain some of their lost weight, few regain it all.

Obesity-related conditions improve: For example, recent research has shown that in obese patients with diabetes, Bariatric surgery resulted in better blood sugar control than medication. This held true no matter what the person weighed before surgery, or how much weight they were able to lose.

Risks and Side Effects

Vomiting: This is a common risk of restrictive surgery caused by the small stomach being overly stretched by food particles that have not been chewed well.

"Dumping syndrome": Caused by malabsorptive surgery, this is when the stomach contents move too rapidly through the small intestine. Symptoms include nausea, weakness, sweating, faintness and, occasionally, diarrhea after eating, as well as the inability to eat sweets, without becoming extremely weak.

Nutritional deficiencies: Patients who have weight loss surgery may develop nutritional deficiencies such as anemia, osteoporosis, and metabolic bone disease. These deficiencies can be avoided if vitamin and mineral intakes are maintained.

Complications: Some patients who have weight loss operations require follow-up operations to correct complications. Complications can include abdominal hernias, infections, breakdown of the staple line (used to make the stomach smaller), and stretched stomach outlets (when the stomach returns to its normal size).

Gallstones: More than 1/3 of obese patients who have gastric surgery develop gallstones. Gallstones are clumps of cholesterol and other matter that forms in the gallbladder. During rapid or substantial weight loss a person's risk of developing gallstones increases. Sometimes this can be prevented by taking supplemental bile salts for the first 6 months after surgery.

Need to temporarily avoid pregnancy: Women of childbearing age should avoid pregnancy until their weight becomes stable because rapid weight loss and nutritional deficiencies can harm a developing fetus.

Side effects: These include nausea, vomiting, bloating, diarrhea, excessive sweating, increased gas, and dizziness.

Lifestyle changes: Patients with extensive bypasses of the normal digestive process require not only close monitoring, but also lifelong diet and exercise modifications and vitamin and mineral supplementation.

Chapter 6: Health Risks of Overweight and Obesity

Being overweight or obese isn't a cosmetic problem. These conditions greatly raise your risk for other health problems.

Coronary Heart Disease:

As your body mass index rises, so does your risk for coronary heart disease (CHD). CHD is a condition in which a waxy substance called plaque (plak) builds up inside the coronary arteries. These arteries supply oxygen-rich blood to your heart.

Plaque can narrow or block the coronary arteries and reduce blood flow to the heart muscle. This can cause angina or a heart attack. (Angina is chest pain or discomfort.)

Obesity can also lead to heart failure. This is a serious condition in which your heart can't pump enough blood to meet your body's needs.

High Blood Pressure:

Blood pressure is the force of blood pushing against the walls of the arteries as the heart pumps blood. If this pressure rises and stays high over time, it can damage the body in many ways.

Your chances of having high blood pressure are greater if you're overweight or obese.

Stroke:

Being overweight or obese can lead to a buildup of plaque in your arteries. Eventually, an area of plaque can rupture, causing a blood clot to form.

If the clot is close to your brain, it can block the flow of blood and oxygen to your brain and cause a stroke. The risk of having a stroke rises as BMI (body mass index) increases.

Type 2 Diabetes:

Diabetes is a disease in which the body's blood glucose or blood sugar level is too high. Normally, the body breaks down food into glucose and then carries it to cells throughout the body. The cells use a hormone called insulin to turn the glucose into energy.

In type 2 diabetes, the body's cells don't use insulin properly. At first, the body reacts by making more insulin. Over time, however, the body can't make enough insulin to control its blood sugar level.

Diabetes is a leading cause of early death, CHD, stroke, kidney disease, and blindness. Most people who have type 2 diabetes are overweight.

Abnormal Blood Fats:

If you're overweight or obese, you're at increased risk of having abnormal levels of blood fats. These include high levels of triglycerides and LDL ("bad") cholesterol and low levels of HDL ("good") cholesterol

Cancer:

Being overweight or obese raises your risk for colon, breast, endometrial, and gallbladder cancers.

Osteoarthritis:

Osteoarthritis is a common joint problem of the knees, hips, and lower back. The condition occurs if the tissue that protects the joints wears away. Extra weight can put more pressure and wear on joints, causing pain.

Sleep Apnea:

Sleep apnea is a common disorder in which you have one or more pauses in breathing or shallow breaths while you sleep.

A person who has sleep apnea may have more fat stored around the neck. This can narrow the airway, making it hard to breathe.

Conclusion

First, understand the basis of weight loss, and think through how you can reduce intake and increase your calorie output.

Then, take out all bad habits: soft drinks, sweets, ice-cream, late night snack and institute good habits and start exercising.

Always try every natural method, before going radical.

If you choose to take medicine, consult your doctor.

Surgery is risky, but maybe the only solution for morbidly obese people.

Make a plan and stick to it.

Remember, YOU CAN DO IT!

www.ingramcontent.com/pod-product-compliance
Lightning Source LLC
Chambersburg PA
CBHW060220290526
45789CB00003B/1344

* 9 7 8 1 5 0 0 9 0 2 6 2 9 *